YOUR KNOWLEDGE HAS VALUE

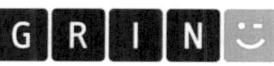

Bibliographic information published by the German National Library:

The German National Library lists this publication in the National Bibliography; detailed bibliographic data are available on the Internet at http://dnb.dnb.de .

Imprint:

Copyright © 2015 GRIN Verlag, Open Publishing GmbH
Print and binding: Books on Demand GmbH, Norderstedt Germany
ISBN: 978-3-668-12549-0

This book at GRIN:

http://www.grin.com/en/e-book/308865/management-functions-of-shaukat-khanum-memorial-cancer-hospital-and-research

Sabir Hussain

Management Functions of Shaukat Khanum Memorial Cancer Hospital and Research. An Analysis

GRIN Publishing

GRIN - Your knowledge has value

Since its foundation in 1998, GRIN has specialized in publishing academic texts by students, college teachers and other academics as e-book and printed book. The website www.grin.com is an ideal platform for presenting term papers, final papers, scientific essays, dissertations and specialist books.

Visit us on the internet:

http://www.grin.com/

http://www.facebook.com/grincom

http://www.twitter.com/grin_com

case study

by Sabir Hussain

13-OCT-2015   WORD COUNT   3006

                     CHARACTER COUNT   16113

A Case study on SKMCH&RC by Sabir Hussain

SHAUKAT KHANUM MEMORIAL CANCER HOSPITAL & RESEARCH CENTRE

1.0   Overview

Shaukat Khanum Memorial Cancer Hospital & Research (SKMCH & RC) is a welfare organization located in Lahore, Pakistan. It is an organizational project by Shaukat Khanum Memorial Trust, which intends to help the poor or ill. It is working in the field of cancer research and treatment. I selected this organization because it is the first and only one organization in Pakistan working at international level in concern of cancer treatment. I took SKMCH & RC as my target case study. This case study has an aim of conducting a review of its management functions and observe how it is working according to international standard. Also, in line with the mission subject, SKMCH & RC has strived hard to remain at the top position of technology. it has done whatever it takes to see that it provides the best quality of technological treatment to patients. The hospital also has an aim of acquiring more medical equipment to see that it fights cancer in the best way possible.

2.0 Introduction

Over the past few years, SKMCH & RC has firmly established itself as a place of excellence providing comprehensive care free of cost to thousands of patients diagnosed with cancer. In September 1985,

Imran Khan, one of Pakistan's most illustrious cricketers, bows to build a cancer hospital in the memory of his mother, Shaukat Khanum, who died from cancer in 1985. January 1990, Dr. Nausherwan Khan Burki draws the master plan. In April 1991 stone lying ceremony conducted by the then Chief Minister of Punjab M. Nawaz Shareef, march 1992 Pakistan wins cricket world cup, a boost to Imran Khan's ambition to build the hospital. In 1992, Leroy Deabler appointed as first hospital director of SKMCH & RC.

In February 1994, mass contact campaign launched with a tour of 30 cities of Pakistan. In February 1995, the hospital has to be thoroughly established, Operation Theater becomes operational for minor surgical, diagnostic and therapeutic procedures. Sui gas and electricity also arrived at the hospital and also first Shaukat Khanum Collection Centre set up at Jail Road, Lahore. Shaukat Khanum has a rigid culture. They have individuals who are cultural oriented and therefore, they ensure they take accounts and decisions in a serious manner.

3.0   Inspiration

Imran Khan and his mother shared a strong bond between them. She was very supportive, and so Imran was so much attached to her. In 1984, Imran's mom, Shaukat Khanum fell sick to a point that once properly diagnosed, she was almost inoperable. She suffered from cancer, which was seeing as a disease which could affect only the rich people, in the sense that only well-off people could afford to fly to Europe where by then most of the treatment was received. It, therefore, saw

1

A Case study on SKMCH&RC by sabir hussain

to be Life style disease. Despite flying to Cromwell Hospital in 1984, Imran's mom died the following year in much pain. Imran made sure that he was by her side all through her hard times. He felt her pain, but he was not in a position to help by any means. In this light, Imran was determined at taking a cancer-related career. When he retired from cricket, he made up his mind to build the first cancer hospital in Pakistan in honor of his mother. SKMCH & RC have a special way of bringing forth innovations. These ways involve encouraging their employees to be risk takers and think of new ideas. They have also bought the idea of decentralization. This means that they have divided the organization into zones. The head of the zone is therefore, expected to borrow ideas from their subordinates while making decisions. They have also invested a lot in guarding the behaviors of the employees. In this therefore, they have formulated rules and regulations that govern employees. For the purpose of meeting organizational objective, SKMCH & RC have gone a notch higher in making sure that they understand what their employees need. They therefore ensure that they motivate their employees through categorizing them. They have also made sure that every employee is given the respect he or she deserves. In this light; therefore, managers are strictly authorized not to use any offense or loose language against the employees. Employees are also motivated through provision of different programs aimed at improving their skills, which in turn would help serve the company in the best way.

4.0 Cancer in Pakistan

Cancer remains to be the major health problem we have today both in developed and developing countries. Statics have shown that in the next two decades the problem of cancer disease will have doubled. Meaning that, in the year 2030, the number of cancer deaths will be about 17 million per year. SKMCH & RC have made it clear to Pakistan citizens that cancer is curable. This is in light to see that people change their misperception they have bout cancer. There exist different religious and cultural myths about cancer. Some people believe that cancer is a death case. In that, once diagnosed with cancer it's impossible for an individual to heal. Laying down the foundation ion of SKMCH & RC was not easy especially now that it was meant to be a cancer centre with expensive medical equipment. such as PET/CT and diagnostic scanners.

In Pakistan, they have provided general statistics concerning cancer cases basing them on the state level. Globecan, 2008 had the following estimates on cancer incidences and mortality in Pakistan as follows.

Cancer incidence was calculated as the weighted average of the observed rates in South Karachi (1998-2002), the Indian estimate and the national estimate for Iran (2008). These data were then applied to the estimated population basing it by sex and age respectively: (i) urban places of the Sindh province (ii) the rural area of Sindh province, Punjab province and Islamabad; (iii) Baluchistan and the North-West Frontier Province (Source: 1998 census).

A Case study on SKMCH&RC by Sabir Hussain

4.1 Mortality

The number of cancer deaths in 2008 was estimated from incidence estimates and site-specific survival, estimated by the GDP method. Some cancer cases and cancer deaths to the estimated World Health Organization had a roughly high number of deaths arising from cancer by sex for 2008.

4.2 Prevalence

The occurrence of cancer was estimated from incidence estimates and the regional average of observed survival by cancer victims and age brackets.

Using this methodology, it is reflected that there are about I SO 000 new cancer cases each year and that between 60% to 80% of these patients have the probability of dying every year. The average age-standardized ratios for cancers victims are 172/ 100 000 for females and 145/ 100 000 for males.

5.0 Initial Fundraisings

On November 10, 1989, Imran Khan made an appeal aimed at collection of funds national wide at Gaddafi Stadium, Lahore, which was able to raise Rs.2,902,600. This was later followed by more than SO potential fundraisers that were held all over the world. Pakistan's win under the leadership of Imran who was by then a captain in the 1992 cricket world cup in Melbourne had a strong effect on fundraising efforts. In the light of the fundraising effect, he was able to collect one and a half million pounds in a successful period of six weeks. This event took place after the world cup. Earlier before the fundraising effect, they had taken a period of two years to raise the same amount. Imran Khan made a contribution of his entire prize money worth of 85,000 pounds for the project. In 1994, Imran's project required much more financing for the construction which was underway. As a result, he, therefore, opted to launch a mass campaign, in which he toured 27 cities in the country and was able to collect Rs. 120 million. During the entire campaign, over a million individual donors ranging from ordinary citizens to the rich and famous showed their willingness and took pa1 1 in the project. Lots of donations were made which aided in the project development. By the virtue that the institute is charitable, it, therefore, depends predominantly on donations made by friends and well-wishers from all over the world. This Organization has a primary goal of developing modern curative measures that will help in eliminating cancer.

6.0 Mission

"To act as an institution which will help in solving the sufferings of patients with cancer by use of modern methods of curative and reduction of pain therapy irrespective of their ability to cater for the expenses, the education of health care professionals, personnel, and the public and to research into the causes, treatment, and preventive measure of cancer".

A Case study on SKMCH&RC by Sabir Hussain

7.0 Vision

7.1 Let's Bowl out Cancer

Imran was a talented all-rounder cricketer and able captain, whose remarkable achievement was leading Pakistan in winning the 1992 World Cup. He uses cricket analogy, and. Therefore, he made a slogan related to a cricket game, and that was Lets Bowl out Cancer.

8.1 UNIQUE ASPECT OF SKMCH SRC ORGANIZATION AND ACHIEVEMENTS

8.1 PET-CT scan

There was no pet ct scan in Pakistan and patients were forced to go abroad for the test. SKMCH and RC, therefore, invested in cyclotron and CT-PET for the benefits of Pakistani patients. This project required a heavy investment of about 5 million us dollar. The organization was able to raise the required amount and henceforth work on the project was initiated, and the facility should be estimated to strut being functional by late 2007.

SKMCH AND RC were able to supply the isotope 18 FOG to other centers as far away as Karachi.

8.2 Bone marrow transplantation

SKMCH AND RC, in the same way, had another great achievement. It was able to conduct its first bone marrow Transplantation procedure on a patient name MUHAMMAD SALMAN on April 26, 2006. This set a record as it was the fourth facility in Pakistan, by the first in

Lahore, to have acquired a bone marrow transplant facility. SKMCH $ RC did not go down on its goals as the transplantation which cost RS 1400000 was conducted free on the patient. The project was finralced by a well-wisher donor whose name remains to be anonymous. This was a big time achievement for the organization as it was able to attain one of the fundamental goals of its foundation. Its goal was to see that it came up with solutions to health issues and make sure that they offer their services to patients at no fee. In this case, we see that its goal was fully accomplished.

9.0 Regular Fundraising

The organization has worked hard to make sure that it mobilizes the public in volunteering itself in matters of financial aid. SKMCH $ RC has therefore come up with various fundraising offices both local and overseas that will help the public reach them in case of an arising issue. The respective office locations include;

9.1 Fundraising Offices

Head Offices, Lahore Regional Offices

Karachi

A Case study on SKMCH&RC by Sabir Hussain

Islamabad

9.2 Overseas Offices

U.K

U.S.A

Gulf

9.3 Sources of funds

The two major sources of fundraising are:

9.3.0 Zakat

9.3.1 Donations

9.3.0 Zakat

On the basis of Shariall (Islamic Rule), an individual has to give about 2.5% of what he owns during the year, in charity, This is referred to as Zakat. It can be offered at any time of the year. Traditionally, most of the people pay Zakat, during the month of Ramadan. To collect maximum amount under the head of Zakat, which is entirely spent on the treatment of poor cancer patients. An intense campaign is carried out in Pakistan and overseas. All offices of SKMCH&RC participate in this activity and are supervised and coordinated by the head office at Lahore.

9.3.1 Donations

The organization carries out campaigns based of fundraising. These campaigns serve an important role in helping facilitate the works of the organization. They can achieve their financial demands through the following types of donations:

Fundraising from Individuals who belongs to the high class

Sponsoring Patients

Concerts

School Campaigns

Equipment / Material Donations

Hide collective donations

10.0   Competitive Analysis

10.1   Challenges/ Threats

Fundraising problems

Healthcare costs/ expenditures

Potential limitation

10.2   Strengths

Free treatment

Developed research centers

Highly-technological equipped machinery

Good check and balances

Preference to quality

10.3   Weaknesses

Lack of government intervention

Sometimes well-wishers might not be reliable

Inadequate skilled personnel

10.4   opportunities

N/A

A Case study on SKMCH&RC by Sabir Hussain

11.0 Competition

Although, SKMCH & RC is not having any such competitor in Asia, if we are to think of any other organization is AGHA KHAN Hospital, which deals with cancer research. SKMCH&RC has the competitive advantage over AGHA KHAN Hospital, in terms of quality treatment and revenue-generating the field. SKMCH & RC has support from some of the well-wishers who help in financing their projects unlike in the case of AGHA KHAN where most of their financial funding must come from their management.

12.0 RESEARCH AT SKMCH&RC

Research at SKMCH&RC is aimed at trying to develop a better understanding of cancer in our society and finding the best solutions of treatment and management of patients in all countries. Overcoming years, their varied knowledge about cancer will have a major impact on our possibility to explain an individual's level of risk of developing cancer. Our ability to examine and diagnose cancer in its early stages and our ability to come up with treatments that is most likely to be effective. We aim to create a connection between the laboratory and clinic through sufficient studies to improve diagnosis, management and prognosis for our cancer patients. The hospital has involved itself in some research work, some of which include cure for cancer and epidemiology studies.

12.1 Research Division Overview

Cancer research is a top priority at SKMCH&RC and has been organized into three different units:-

The Clinical Research Office, an active clinical trials office involved in several international studies from major pharmaceutical companies. Data from clinical trials of drugs used to treat cancer worldwide enables us to evaluate the dose, duration and effectiveness of treatment for our patients.

Cancer Registry and Clinical Data Management (CRCDM) unit and Disease-Specific Registry are responsible for maintaining the hospital-based cancer registry, compiling a disease-specific index (cancerous and non-cancerous) using international classification systems on all cancer/non-cancer patients registered and/or treated at this hospital, and running the disease-specific projects. It generates cancer statistics from the registry database using an advanced medical records system, a part of the hospital information system. To enhance its studies in the epidemiology of cancers, the unit is attempting to develop a population-based city-wide cancer registry with the help of other hospitals and laboratories within the city of Lahore. The regist1-y has also been involved in conducting a pilot project on breast cancer screening in a locality close to the hospital.

The Basic Science Research Laboratory is equipped to conduct various intense studies, some of which include molecular, cellular, and genetic. The lab is involved in efforts of trying to acquire information about the genetic and environmental factor that cause cancers in Pakistan, through combined epidemiological studies. Specific viruses have also been associated with cancer. Intense studies are being conducted to determine the role of known

6

A Case study on SKMCH&RC by Sabir Hussain

pathogens in cancer development in our population, with the hope that effective preventative measures will reduce the number of cases. The immunology and pathogenesis of a variety of cancers are currently being examined through some research works by the research scientists of SKMCH&RC. This is with an aim to come up with better ways to diagnose cancer at early stages and to monitor the effectiveness of treatment over the diagnosed period.

13.0   Criticism

Although there is no documented proof of corruption on SKMCH&RC, it is still subjected to criticisms. SKMCH&RC faces lots of false allegations from the public. It also faces political challenges because its founder has become a political figure.

13.1   Current statement of CEO on accounts criticism

The CEO SKMCH&RC has denied any financial irregularity and embezzlement of funds in its activities.

While in a press conference, SKMCH&RC CEO Dr. Faisal Sultan stated that the hospital was an internationally recognized institution, formed and still managed by the help and support of the people of Pakistan.

He said that criticism on hospital's endowment fund was baseless as all the financial matters of the hospital were documented and were available on its website for public. He said that the SKMCH&RC funds have been invested with positive intentions and are safe. He added that the hospital's accounts were audited by internationally acclaimed firms.

He said that SKMCH&RC has played a major role in the treatment of cancer patients who are not well up and had spent more than Rs 10 billion in this regard. That was why international organizations like the World Health Organization appreciated the hospital's role and the Royal College of Physicians, Edinburgh, awarded an honorally fellowship to Imran Khan.

Dr. Sultan added that 75 percent of patients at SKMCH&RC got financial support and the number was increasing, adding that the budget of the hospital increases every year. "By the support of the people, we manage the increased budget. It's only because the people have faith in this hospital, and we will try to maintain their trust as long as we live," he said.

He also said that SKMCH&RC was not Imran Khan's personal property, it was a public entity, and the Pakistani nation owned it. While talking about the plans, he said that a complete cancer hospital in Peshawar and another one in Karachi were in planning process. He acknowledged the role of the media for its support and hoped that this support would continue in the future as well.

SKMCH&RC has its management and business process at a high notch. The organization makes sure that it implements each and evely goal it sets. They are self driven and therefore no cases of discrimination amongst themselves. They follow up their rules and regulations as stipulated in their company's Statement. In the same way, SKMCH&RC makes evaluation of their performance at regular intervals. In case of any deviation from what is expected, they make sure that they take the appropriate action.

A Case study on SKMCH&RC by Sabir Hussain

14.0   References

https://ww.shaukatkhanum.org.pk/component/content/article/18-imran-khan.html

https://www.shaukatkhanum.org.pk/how-to-help/426.html

http://jjco.oxfordjournals.org/content/43/8/771.full

http://archives.dailytimes.com.pk/national/23-Nov-2003/skmch-gets-new-radition-equipment

http://www.shaukatkhanum.org.pk/research.html

http://archives.dailytimes.com.pk/lahore/04-Aug-2012/no-irregulatities-in-accounts-skmch

8

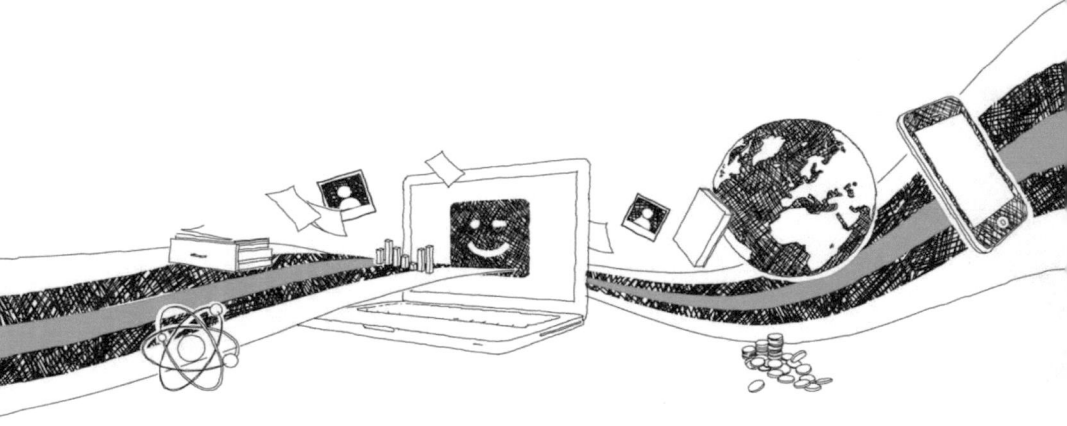
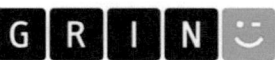